HEALED

THE MYSTERY OF DIVINE HEALING

THE HEALING SERIES
BOOK 1

CHAD GONZALES

ISBN: 979-8-9916262-0-0

Copyright © 2024 by Chad Gonzales

All rights reserved.

No part of this book may be reproduced in any form or by any electronic or mechanical means, including information storage and retrieval systems, without written permission from the author, except for the use of brief quotations in a book review.

CONTENTS

1. Prophetic Insight — 1
2. Jesus Became Sick — 7
3. The Relationship Between Sin and Sickness — 11
4. The Day You Died to Sickness — 17
5. Healed From the Source — 21
6. Raising Up The Dead Man — 25

About the Author — 29
Also by Chad Gonzales — 31
The Healing Academy — 33

1 PROPHETIC INSIGHT

One of the most well-known scriptures in the Bible regarding healing is 1 Peter 2:24. If you have heard teaching on healing, I can almost guarantee you have heard this scripture mentioned. In fact, it is one of the few scriptures written to the Church that specifically mentions physical healing. There has been an exhaustive amount of teaching on it, especially since the early 1900s. Unfortunately, we have only scratched the surface of what it is really about, and as a result, it has left people in frustration.

Some have taught that Peter is only talking about spiritual healing; others have taught that it is about physical healing; and yet others have taught that it's about physical healing when you die and go to Heaven. The purpose of this book is to take the complexity out of all of this and help you see the beautiful reality of what Jesus actually provided for us in this one wonderful scripture.

I have been on a journey for the last twenty-plus years of studying and teaching in the area of divine healing. Revelation is certainly progressive, and I can say that in my own growth, my understanding of healing has continued to grow as I have pursued understanding and wisdom in this area. For the longest time, I never really touched on what we would call the redemptive scriptures on healing, such as Isaiah 53:4-5, Matthew 8:17, and 1 Peter 2:24.

> **Isaiah 53:4-5 (NKJV)**: "Surely He has borne our griefs and carried our sorrows; yet we esteemed Him stricken, smitten by God, and afflicted. But He was wounded for our transgressions, He was bruised for our iniquities; the chastisement for our peace was upon Him, and by His stripes we are healed."

> **Matthew 8:17 (NKJV)**: "...that it might be fulfilled which was spoken by Isaiah the prophet, saying: 'He Himself took our infirmities and bore our sicknesses.'"

> **1 Peter 2:24 (NKJV)**: "...who Himself bore our sins in His own body on the tree, that we,

having died to sins, might live for righteousness—by whose stripes you were healed."

For almost two decades, I have taught healing strictly from the standpoint of our union and identity with Christ. The result was that I taught from the book of John, looking at Jesus' union with the Father and the "In Christ" scriptures found in the apostle Paul's letters to the churches, such as Romans, Ephesians, Galatians, and Colossians.

Last year, the Holy Spirit led me to go back and look at these three passages of scripture. Because of my continued focus and foundation of our union with Christ, these three passages of scripture came alive to me like never before, especially 1 Peter 2:24.

If you were to ask the average Christian what 1 Peter 2:24 says, most would say, "By the stripes of Jesus, I was healed." Although that is part of the scripture, it is not the entire verse. Let's read it in its entirety:

1 Peter 2:24 (NKJV): "Who Himself bore our sins in His own body on the tree, that we, having died to sins, might live for righteousness—by whose stripes you were healed."

What we have here is a beautiful statement of redemption that is so simple and yet profound—only the Holy Spirit could write it. And yet, Peter was simply quoting what the Holy Spirit showed the prophet Isaiah over 700 years prior.

> **Isaiah 53:5 (NKJV)**: "But He was wounded for our transgressions, He was bruised for our iniquities; the chastisement for our peace was upon Him, and by His stripes we are healed."

To fully understand the true meaning of 1 Peter 2:24, we need to understand what Isaiah was talking about. In Isaiah 53, we find Isaiah prophesying about the future coming of the Messiah. God supernaturally allowed Isaiah to see, in real time, something that wouldn't happen for over 700 years. God showed Jesus dying for us. However, what is interesting is that Isaiah isn't seeing the physical side—Isaiah is seeing the spiritual side.

Almost all of the focus on Jesus on the cross is centered on Jesus being physically tortured, whipped, the crown of thorns placed on His head, and nailed to a cross. It was one of the most gruesome and horrendous deaths someone could face, but it was even worse on the spiritual side. If we could have seen spiritually what was happening that day, no Hollywood horror movie could match it. God had given Isaiah insight into what was happening spiritually, just as God had shown David prophetically about 1,000 years before.

> **Psalm 22:1, 12-18 (AMPC)**: "My God, my God, why have You forsaken me? Why are You so far from helping me, and from the words of my groaning? ... Many [foes like] bulls have surrounded me; strong bulls of Bashan have hedged me in. ... For [like a pack of] dogs they have encompassed me; a company of evildoers has encircled me, they pierced my hands and my feet. ... They part my clothing among them and cast lots for my raiment (a long, shirtlike garment, a seamless undertunic)."

Like Isaiah, David was prophetically seeing Jesus and the cross. David describes mostly the physical, but there is a reason Jesus cried out on the cross, "My God, my God, why have You forsaken Me!" The reason was simple: the physical pain was horrible, but the spiritual pain was worse because Jesus had become sin.

2 JESUS BECAME SICK

Jesus became sin. Now, please understand: Jesus was not a sinner. JESUS NEVER SINNED AND WAS NOT A SINNER; however, He became sin and became sick. This prophetic insight by Isaiah reveals several things.

> **Isaiah 53:4-5 (AMPC)**: "Surely He has borne our griefs (sicknesses, weaknesses, and distresses) and carried our sorrows and pains [of punishment], yet we [ignorantly] considered Him stricken, smitten, and afflicted by God [as if with leprosy]. But He was wounded for our transgressions, He was bruised for our guilt and iniquities; the chastisement [needful to obtain] peace and well-being for us was upon Him, and with the stripes [that

wounded] Him we are healed and made whole."

The word *griefs* is the Hebrew word *choliy,* which literally and simply means "sickness." The word *sorrows* is the Hebrew word *mak'ob,* which literally and simply means "physical and emotional pains." It is crystal clear that Isaiah is speaking of Jesus bearing our physical issues in verse 4. In the same way Jesus became sin, Jesus became sickness; there is no way around this.

Isaiah goes on to say that the chastisement of our peace was upon Him. The word *peace* is the Hebrew word *shalowm,* which is fascinating. It means "completeness, soundness, welfare, peace, prosperity, health, and peace from war." The word *healed* is the Hebrew word *rapha,* which means "healing" or "physician."

Here again, we see that "by His stripes, we are healed" is unequivocally talking about physical healing. Jesus bore our punishment so that we can be free of sickness and disease. Jesus not only became sin; as a result, Jesus also became sickness so that we could be free spiritually, mentally, and physically.

Isaiah goes on in verse 10 and reveals a staggering truth.

Isaiah 53:10 (NKJV): "Yet it pleased the Lord to bruise Him; He has put Him to grief. When You make His soul an offering for sin, He shall see His seed, He shall prolong His days, and the pleasure of the Lord shall prosper in His hand."

Do you see what this says?

It pleased God to bruise Him and put Him to grief because Jesus became an offering for our sin! The word *bruise* is the Hebrew word *daka,* which means "to be crushed." The word *grief* is the Hebrew word *chalah,* which means…are you ready? *Chalah* means "to be made sick."

Look at this. It was God Himself who placed the crushing weight of sin on Jesus, and yet we are also blatantly told that Jesus was made to be sick as well. Jesus became sick in the same way He became sin. Why did it please God to do this? From a physical side, it seems grossly horrific that a loving father would be pleased to do this to His child—but this is where we err. We must always see what's going on from the spiritual side, and this is what Isaiah was showing us. Jesus was the righteous Son of God, but He also became the spotless, sacrificial Lamb to be the sacrifice for our sin and the seed of faith sown by God to reap a harvest of many sons and daughters.

In looking at Isaiah's prophecy, we see without question that Jesus became the sacrifice for our sicknesses, and thus it reveals God's will for our healing. God made Jesus sick because He didn't want us sick! Not only do we see God's absolute will for our physical healing and the sacrifice of Jesus for it, but we also see something else—a relationship between sin and sickness.

When we begin to look at the spiritual side of things, we can see cause and effect. We see that sickness was the result of sin, and this is why when Jesus became sin, He became sick; yet the bearing of our sin was also the bearing of our sickness. There is always cause and effect. Where you see sickness, you will find sin—but it's not in the way you probably are thinking right now. There is a relationship between sin and sickness that must be understood.

3 THE RELATIONSHIP BETWEEN SIN AND SICKNESS

Sickness and disease never showed up until sin showed up. When God made the earth, it was perfect. However, when Adam and Eve sinned, it released the curse into the world. As a result, sickness came. You could say that sin was the root of the problem, and sickness was a fruit of the root. It was the sin of Adam that released sickness into the world for all of humanity.

Throughout Scripture, we see the relationship between sin and sickness. There are several stories in the Gospel accounts that reveal this connection, but in my opinion, there is none greater than the story of the paralyzed man who was brought to Jesus.

> **Luke 5:17-25 (NKJV)**: "Now it happened on a certain day, as He was teaching, that there

were Pharisees and teachers of the law sitting by, who had come out of every town of Galilee, Judea, and Jerusalem. And the power of the Lord was present to heal them. Then behold, men brought on a bed a man who was paralyzed, whom they sought to bring in and lay before Him. And when they could not find how they might bring him in, because of the crowd, they went up on the housetop and let him down with his bed through the tiling into the midst before Jesus. When He saw their faith, He said to him, 'Man, your sins are forgiven you.' And the scribes and the Pharisees began to reason, saying, 'Who is this who speaks blasphemies? Who can forgive sins but God alone?' But when Jesus perceived their thoughts, He answered and said to them, 'Why are you reasoning in your hearts? Which is easier, to say, "Your sins are forgiven you," or to say, "Rise up and walk"? But that you may know that the Son of Man has power on earth to forgive sins'—He said to the man who was paralyzed, 'I say to you, arise, take up your bed, and go to your house.' Immediately he rose up before them, took up what he had been lying on, and departed to his own house, glorifying God. And they were all amazed,

THE RELATIONSHIP BETWEEN SIN AND SICKNESS 13

and they glorified God and were filled with fear, saying, 'We have seen strange things today!'"

Did you notice what Jesus said to the paralyzed man when he was dropped through the roof? Jesus said, "Man, your sins are forgiven you." That seems like an odd thing to say to someone who needs healing! But Jesus understood the covenant the Israelites had with God, and He also understood the root cause of all sickness and disease: sin.

Jesus isn't dealing with the fruit of the problem; Jesus is going straight after the root of the problem. Do you know why Jesus said, "You are forgiven?" Because Jesus understood that when you cut off the root, you automatically kill off the fruit. Fruit can't grow on a tree when the roots of the tree are removed.

The Israelites knew that in their covenant, as long as they didn't sin, they didn't get sick; this was their covenant with God. If you keep sin out, you keep sickness out. So when Jesus told the man that he was forgiven, Jesus was essentially saying, "You are healed." The problem was that the man and the Pharisees didn't understand. This is why Jesus went on to say, "Which is easier, to say, 'Your sins are forgiven you,' or to say, 'Rise up and walk?'" Jesus was revealing the relationship between sin and sickness. When Jesus healed him, Jesus was also revealing the man was forgiven. When you remove the root, you automatically remove the fruit; sin was the source, and sickness was the byproduct.

Now, before we go any further, I don't want you thinking that if you are sick, or a close friend or loved one is sick, it is because they have sinned. We will get into that in just a bit; but we must understand that the reason sickness is in the earth is because of sin. Essentially, sin and sickness are the same. When we see the word *sin,* we can substitute it with the word *sickness.* And when we understand the spiritual side of sickness, it opens our eyes to wonderful truths hidden within Scripture that are actually meant to be openly revealed.

> **2 Corinthians 5:21 (NKJV)**: "For He made Him who knew no sin to be sin for us, that we might become the righteousness of God in Him."

Substitute the word *sin* with *sickness* and read it like this: "He made Him who knew no sickness to be sickness for us, that we might become the righteousness of God in Him." Isn't that amazing? And yet, this is exactly what Isaiah saw! God made Jesus sin and sickness so that we become righteous.

Wait…do you see this? Is it possible that righteousness has more to do with just "being forgiven?" Absolutely it does. Righteousness is more than just being forgiven and being in a good position with God; righteousness is also about being healed.

4 THE DAY YOU DIED TO SICKNESS

In Romans 6, the Apostle Paul gives a great mini-teaching on redemption. There are powerful truths here about our identity and union with Christ and the realities of what Jesus did for us.

> **Romans 6:4-11 (NKJV):** 4 Therefore we were buried with Him through baptism into death, that just as Christ was raised from the dead by the glory of the Father, even so we also should walk in newness of life. 5 For if we have been united together in the likeness of His death, certainly we also shall be in the likeness of His resurrection, 6 knowing this, that our old man was crucified with Him, that the body of sin might be done away with, that we should no longer be slaves of sin. 7 For he who has died

has been freed from sin. 8 Now if we died with Christ, we believe that we shall also live with Him, 9 knowing that Christ, having been raised from the dead, dies no more. Death no longer has dominion over Him. 10 For the death that He died, He died to sin once for all; but the life that He lives, He lives to God. 11 Likewise you also, reckon yourselves to be dead indeed to sin, but alive to God in Christ Jesus our Lord.

Notice in Romans 6:4, we are told that we were buried with Christ and raised with Christ so we would experience the same life as Christ. Paul is teaching on union and identity here. In verses 6-7, we are told that Jesus made us dead to sin. How is that possible? Because the death that Jesus died is the death we died! What Jesus died to, we died to! What Jesus was made alive unto, we were made alive unto!

2 Corinthians 5:17, 21 (NKJV) : 17 Therefore, if anyone is in Christ, he is a new creation; old things have passed away; behold, all things have become new. 21 For He made Him who knew no sin to be sin for us, that we might become the righteousness of God in Him.

When Jesus died with sin and sickness, it died with Him. Jesus took the root of the problem and killed it. It was the day that sin and sickness died.

The day you made Jesus your Lord and Savior is the day the old you died and a new life began. This new life is a righteous life; it's a life of being dead to sin and no longer being a slave. The root of sin was cut off, and we died to it. Righteousness is more than just a good position with God. Righteousness is about being forgiven, but not just forgiven of sin—dead to sin…and dead to sickness. So we could read Romans 6:6-7 like this:

Romans 6:6-7 (author's rendition) - 6 knowing this, that our old man was crucified with Him, that the body of sickness might be done away with, that we should no longer be slaves of sickness. 7 For he who has died has been freed from sickness.

The old me died. When the old me died, the one that was a slave to sickness died. How is that possible? Because the sin problem was removed. When I died, I died to sin, and as a result of the root being dead, the fruit died too.

5 HEALED FROM THE SOURCE

With all of these truths established, let's take a fresh look at 1 Peter 2:24 and discover what this is really all about.

> **1 Peter 2:24 (AMPC):** He personally bore our sins in His [own] body on the tree [as on an altar and offered Himself on it], that we might die (cease to exist) to sin and live to righteousness. By His wounds you have been healed.

First, remember that Peter is quoting Isaiah, and we know unequivocally that Isaiah was talking about physical healing in Isaiah 53. Well, if Isaiah was talking about physical healing, then 1 Peter 2:24 is referring to physical healing as well.

A majority of people have viewed 1 Peter 2:24 in regards to spiritual healing. First of all, there is no such thing as "spiritual healing." You can't heal your spirit; the spirit of man must be born again. Once you are born again, there is nothing to be healed. However, there is a tiny bit of truth in that this is a spiritual thing, and this is where Christians get hung up on this verse. Disease is a spiritual thing. How is that possible? Because sin is a spiritual thing. Well, if sin is the root and sickness is the fruit, if one is spiritual, the other has to be spiritual too. So, sickness is a spiritual thing.

Secondly, Peter is not telling us something we need to get. Peter is telling us who we are. In reality, 1 Peter 2:24 is not a healing scripture; it is a righteousness scripture! It is telling us WHO WE ARE, not WHAT WE NEED TO GET.

The prophet Isaiah was looking into the future and seeing Jesus in the present; Isaiah said, "By His stripes we are healed." Peter is looking back and seeing what happened to Jesus in the past! This is why Peter says, "by His stripes, you WERE HEALED." This is a done deal.

Now here is the big piece I need you to get. I want you to truly understand what is meant by "You were healed." For centuries, we have been taught that this was about healing your body of disease. Although the healing of disease is there, it is more than that. Jesus didn't just heal you of the problem; Jesus healed you of the source! Jesus didn't just remove the fruit; Jesus removed the root! Before you were connected to sin, there was a flow of sickness into your life—but then Jesus came and healed you! Jesus healed you from sin, and as a result, Jesus healed you from sickness.

Do you see the connection? Jesus bore our sins. When Jesus died, we died. Through death, we cease to exist to sin. Now remember, sin is the root of the problem. Without sin, there is no sickness; they are a package deal. As a result of sin being removed, we are the righteousness of God. Because we are righteous, forgiven, and dead to sin, we are healed.

"By His stripes, you are healed" is not just removing you from the problem; it is removing you from the source of the problem. When you died to sin, you died to disease! You need to start going through life and every time you hear about a sickness, say, "I'm dead to it!"

We need to stop trying to get healed. We need to stop asking God to heal us. We need to stop waiting on God to manifest it. These things are not new creation realities, and they are not to be even in the mindset of the new creation.

How can God give you what He already gave you?

How can God give you what He already made you?

You are the righteousness of God in Christ. In Christ, you are righteous, perfect, and complete. If you are righteous, you are healed. Why? Because if you are righteous, you are forgiven. If you are righteous, you are dead to sin. If you are dead to sin, you are dead to disease. Case closed.

6 RAISING UP THE DEAD MAN

So then the logical question is, "If I am dead to sickness, then why do I still experience it?" Are you ready? It's not because of your works; it is because of your imaginations.

> **Colossians 2:8-14 (NKJV):** 8 Beware lest anyone cheat you through philosophy and empty deceit, according to the tradition of men, according to the basic principles of the world, and not according to Christ. 9 For in Him dwells all the fullness of the Godhead bodily; 10 and you are complete in Him, who is the head of all principality and power. 11 In Him you were also circumcised with the circumcision made without hands, by putting off the body of the sins of the flesh, by the

circumcision of Christ, 12 buried with Him in baptism, in which you also were raised with Him through faith in the working of God, who raised Him from the dead. 13 And you, being dead in your trespasses and the uncircumcision of your flesh, He has made alive together with Him, having forgiven you all trespasses, 14 having wiped out the handwriting of requirements that was against us, which was contrary to us. And He has taken it out of the way, having nailed it to the cross.

What is the possibility that the only reason we still see sickness is because we think it is still possible for dead people? What is the possibility that the only reason we continue to get sick is because we keep resurrecting the dead man?

We are buried with Christ. The old man that was a slave to sin and sickness died with Christ. The problem is, we keep raising that dead man up from the grave. How? Because we still think it's possible to get sick. The moment we start looking at what the world calls normal, we begin to identify with the sinner once again. You may be saved and going to Heaven, but the moment you start identifying with the sinner, you'll start experiencing the results of the sinner.

If you think sickness is normal, sickness will be normal for you. How? You raised up the old you, identified with the old you, and are trying to live like the old you.

This is why the apostle Paul tells us to renew our minds!

> **Romans 12:2 (NKJV)**: 2 And do not be conformed to this world, but be transformed by the renewing of your mind, that you may prove what is that good and acceptable and perfect will of God.

> **Colossians 3:1-3 (NKJV)**: If then you were raised with Christ, seek those things which are above, where Christ is, sitting at the right hand of God. 2 Set your mind on things above, not on things on the earth. 3 For you died, and your life is hidden with Christ in God.

If we do not start seeing ourselves according to who we are in Christ and what is normal for Christ, we will still live like a sinner while going to Heaven. Now, I didn't say you are a sinner. You don't have to sin to live like a sinner. You can think like a sinner and live like a sinner because you still have the perspective of the sinner.

We can't think like the dead man anymore. We can't see like the dead man anymore. We must see ourselves like the new creation in Christ that we are. We must see ourselves as righteous, forgiven, complete, perfect, and healed. Stop identifying as the old man alive to sickness and identify with Jesus as dead to sickness and alive to God. Now, because of your union with Christ, whatever is flowing in Him is flowing in you. If sickness can't flow in Him, it can't flow in you—because you are dead to sin.

Healing for the body is not based on your works; healing for the body is based on Jesus removing you from the source of sickness: sin.

All throughout the Scripture, this is the marvelous truth regarding healing. Healing is the byproduct of righteousness. When you remove sin, you remove sickness. Jesus didn't come to just heal you of the problem; Jesus came to heal you of the source!

By the stripes of Jesus, you were healed!

ABOUT THE AUTHOR

Chad Gonzales, founder of The Healing Academy, is a visionary leader dedicated to helping individuals unlock their divine potential and experience miraculous healings through a deep commitment to Jesus Christ's teachings. With extensive education in counseling and theology, Chad combines profound knowledge with practical experience from over two decades as a pastor and church planter.

As a prolific author, his latest book, "The Supernatural Prayer of Jesus," empowers readers to tap into the extraordinary power of faith. Chad continues to inspire believers globally through his teachings, programs, and media platforms. He is a living testament to the miraculous possibilities that await those who dare to believe, leaving an indelible mark on their spiritual journeys.

chadgonzales.com

ALSO BY CHAD GONZALES

Advance

Advance: The Devotional

Aliens

An Alternate Reality

Believing God For A House

Eight Percent

Fearless

God's Will Is You Healed

Making Right Decisions

Naturally Supernatural

The Freedom of Forgiveness

The Supernatural Prayer of Jesus

Think Like Jesus

Walking In The Miraculous

What's Next

THE HEALING ACADEMY

The Healing Academy is an outreach of Chad Gonzales Ministries to help the everyday believer learn to walk according to the standard of Jesus in the ministry of healing. Jesus said in John 14:12 that whoever believes in Him would do the same works and even greater works. Through The Healing Academy, it is our goal to raise the standard of the healing ministry in the Church and manifest the ministry of Jesus in the marketplace. For more information, please visit thehealingacademy.com

Made in the USA
Middletown, DE
27 February 2025